If It Fits Y

The Ultimate Guide to IIFYM Flexible Dieting: Burn Fat, Gain Energy and Build Muscle

~ Katherine Wright

CONTENTS

Introduction

Chapter 1 – Food Battle: Healthy vs. Unhealthy

Chapter 2 – Avoiding Nutritional Excess and Deficiency

Chapter 3 – Healthy Diet vs. IIFYM Diet Plan

Chapter 4 – Achieving Macronutrient Balance

Conclusion

Check Out My Other Books

If It Fits Your Macros: Copyright © 2016 by LFI Publishing All rights reserved. No part of this book may be reproduced in any form without permission in writing from the author. Reviewers may quote brief passages in reviews.

Disclaimer

No part of this publication may be reproduced or transmitted in any form or by any means, mechanical or electronic, including photocopying or recording, or by any information storage and retrieval system, or transmitted by email without permission in writing from the publisher.

While all attempts have been made to verify the information provided in this publication, neither the author nor the publisher assumes any responsibility for errors, omissions, or contrary interpretations of the subject matter herein.

This book is for informational purposes only. The views expressed are those of the author alone, and should not be taken as expert instruction or commands. The reader is responsible for his or her own actions. The advice and strategies contained in this book may not even be suitable for your situation, and you should consult your own advisors as appropriate.

Adherence to all applicable laws and regulations, including international, federal, state, and local governing professional licensing, business practices, advertising, and all other aspects of doing business in the US, Canada, or any other jurisdiction is the sole responsibility of the purchaser or reader.

Neither the author nor the publisher assumes any responsibility or liability whatsoever on the behalf of the purchaser or reader of these materials.

Any perceived slight of any individual or organization is purely unintentional.

Introduction

Hi, my name is Katy Wright. I'm a food lover and a health nut. I got into the world of fitness and health when I was pretty young and I've tried a lot of different things out. You could call me a bit of a human guinea pig when it comes to diets. My hope is to pass on some of my findings so I can help others attain their perfect body and better health.

I'll first get this out of the way, even though it's covered in my disclaimer: before starting any diet, speak to your doctor or appropriate licensed medical practitioner. Okay, done with that, now onto the good stuff.

I love that you picked up my book, "If It Fits Your Macros". I have a variety of books on the subject of losing weight but I have found that the diet that's easiest to follow and gets the best results is the one that you can stick to. Whether that's low carb, paleo, vegetarian etc. As long as you feel comfortable eating the foods you're making or ordering and you can do it every day, that's what's going to work. Personally I like eating bacon so I enjoy any type of diet lifestyle that lets me enjoy my favorite food.

Yes, you heard me, lots of bacon; and that's not all. After trying a dizzying array of diets and supplements I can honestly say that being able to indulge in all your favorite "bad foods" is one of the best ways to maintain a healthy body and slim down. I know you're probably thinking that it's counterintuitive to eat fat and be healthy, but the tides have been turning lately and the evidence is piling up. Whether you're a fan of South Beach or the Paleo diet or you've only heard of the Atkins diet, this book has got real information for real results.

If It Fits Your Macros is a diet name that has really just started to gain traction and in many ways it's flexible style is more similar to "clean eating." This happens to be a bit of a dirty word in the eyes of the IIFYM crowd though. So I'll get into the true nitty gritty of IIFYM and you can decide if it's for you.

You'll find in the following pages some sage advice on how and why you should be giving the low carb and high fat diet a try. If you're looking for long lasting results, you won't just "diet" you'll change your lifestyle. By adjusting your diet to be more flexible and sticking to your macro ingredients you'll get the body you want and love and the health to enjoy it for a lot longer.

Thanks again for downloading this book, I hope you enjoy it!

Chapter 1 – Food Battle: Healthy vs. Unhealthy

There's something wrong in assigning indiscriminate "percentages of important" on the specific components of a person's fitness regimen. This includes the popular yet unproven statement "Your fitness is determined by 10% exercise and 90% diet." For the time being, let's just agree on the value of nutrition as a primary aspect of your health. Now that we have this large portion of the pie on your plate, you still need to sort out another challenge – how much of your nutrition is composed of clean/healthy diet and how much is dirty/unhealthy?

Let's assume that you have apple pie on the table. Now look at the pie. Surely, apples contain lots of nutritional value, which means apples are clean. So you can eat only the apples. But what about that sweet, gooey filling that holds the apples together? All that sugar and water that brings you a piece of heaven every time you take a bit.

How about that tasty and crunchy crust that smells so good? Is this part of the apple pie unhealthy for you?

The Significance of Being Healthy?

Honestly, there's no straightforward answer for the questions mentioned above, because being "healthy" is applicable to your own unique nutritional needs. People have the tendency to arbitrarily tag the word "healthy" around in specific pre-outlined conditions. However, what is considered healthy for one person may not be healthy for another. Following the Darwinian principles of evolution, for something to be healthy, it should improve the survivability or fitness of that living thing.

Extreme Diets Are Not Effective In the Long Run

Usually, diets that offer impractical provisions or significantly limit specific nutrients are not sustainable for the long-term because of the strict demands and inclination towards imbalance. A more doable diet, on the other hand, is much easier to stick to. No matter how great a diet regimen appears on paper, it will never work if it is impractical. Remember, the human body is a breathing, living being and not a piece of machine. Today, physique sports and bodybuilding encourage extreme routine and diet, and as a matter of fact this resulted to the entire dichotomy of "healthy" and "unhealthy" foods.

People who are into "healthy" regimen, examine specific food and think "Nuts, vegetables, and fish, are all "clean" foods, so I will only follow a meal plan composed mostly of these foods, and stay away from those that are not healthy.

What Makes a Food Healthy or Unhealthy?

Let's stop for a few moments and think about it sensibly. What makes, for instance, a piece of smoked red herring with lemon "healthy?" Is it the protein content, given that an average serving could provide you with 19.6 grams of protein? Probably it is "healthy" because of its omega-3 content that as proven by science could help you prevent heart diseases.

In the same line of thinking, how can we define a certain type of food as "unhealthy"? I'm certain that you are now thinking of foods such as burger, ice cream, potato chips, pizza, fries whenever you encounter the phrase "unhealthy food". How can we say that they are "unhealthy"? Is it because these foods are processed, high in sugar or fat, and insufficient in important nutrients?

By now, you might be overwhelmed with a lot of questions, but you must not worry as you can find answers in the following sections and chapters.

The Relevance of IIFYM Diet

The diet known as IIFYM (If It Fits Your Macros) has started to gain ground as a dieting regimen, especially in the bodybuilding niche. However, this diet is not really a new or intense regimen. As a matter of fact, IIFYM is unofficially the method used by people who has ever monitored their food intake with the exclusion that there is no restriction in the types of food allowed. Certainly, in the fitness and bodybuilding world, the concept of no foods being restricted has sent many "health" fanatics into a rage, dismissing IIFYM as being a mediocre and irrational way of dieting. This could be surprising for some readers, mostly those who have been following a type of extreme diet for years. But in reality, very few types of foods are generally unhealthy and totally unfavorable to your overall health and wellness.

Prohibiting certain food allergies or an unreasonable fear of particular food additives such as monosodium glutamate, there's no solid basis to tag a food as being completely unhealthy.

The Risk Is On the Toxicity

Now before you react negatively on the notion described above, you should know that there are lots of research that goes into the possible damaging effects of artificial food ingredients as well as additives. But practically, it's unreasonable to worry about being unhealthy if you are not consuming these things every day in overwhelming quantities. Great examples include are high-fructose corn syrup and partially hydrogenated oils. These food ingredients have received bad reputation, particularly with their increasing use in the food supply and the associated rise in the number of people who are obese.

It is true that trans-fat produced from partially hydrogenated oils could increase the risk for heart complications even in small quantities. But if you are only consuming less than a gram of trans-fat every day, which is not that difficult to make sure unless you plan on munching cakes every minute, then the health complications are trivial.

And in the defense of high-fructose corn syrup, you can avoid health complications if you limit your intake. But practically, if you are consuming an otherwise healthy diet and you care regulating your calorie intake, a small amount of high-fructose corn syrup will not cause a detrimental effect on your health or physique.

Unfortunately, promoting the moderation principles of IIFYM to a crowd of fitness aficionados and bodybuilding fanatics possibly will not bode well for the reception of this book, but this is really a great transition into the next chapter that will examine the few pitfalls of the IIFYM principles and how you can rectify them.

Chapter 2 – Avoiding Nutritional Excess and Deficiency

In the first Chapter of this book, we have discussed a few things that make a certain diet or food healthy or unhealthy, and how there is no generic formula out there that will provide you with certain nutritional needs.

It is recommended that you take time to understand the specific metabolic requirements of your body. You can do this more likely through trial and error. But the primary thing to keep in mind is that any natural diet that can help you optimize your performance must be avoiding the extremes of consuming too much of a certain nutrient and taking insufficient level of another nutrient as well as meeting your everyday calorie requirement.

Remember, regardless of the types of food that you want to eat, a diet is only a tool to achieve your desired results. This is the essence of IIFYM.

But one of the main flaws of IIFYM is that some people use this diet as an excuse to ignore things such as dietary fibers, micronutrients, essential fatty acids, protein, and sugar.

For instance, a diet composed of too much soy protein will possibly not be effective for muscle building and fat loss compared to a diet composed of high-quality protein, particularly rich in leucine such as whey and egg whites.

So What Really Is IIFYM?

Macro refers to macronutrients, of which there are four types: protein, carbohydrates, fat, and alcohol. Also added is one consideration: fiber. It is an important component of carbohydrates macronutrients, although some of those in the nutrition company regard fiber as a micro nutrient. In this book, we will refer to fiber intake as an important consideration when dieting, so I have included it with the other macros.

IIFYM is specifically designed for fat loss through macro nutrition and hence a caloric perspective and is absolutely a tool to improve nutritional composition of the body. It is not designed to address health issues of the brain, heart, or other body organs and it is not promoted as a type of a healthy diet.

Whether you want to ear cheese burger or spinach pecan salad, IIFYM advocates the notion that eating less calories below your body requirement while still getting enough protein, carbohydrates, fat, and fiber based on your targets and the energy requirements of your body, you can boost weight loss. IIFYM is an easy tool to lose weight. You just need to stay within your everyday macros and you can easily get rid of fat.

IIFYM Origins

IIFYM was arbitrarily initiated by several bodybuilders who grew tired of eating boring food when they were preparing for bodybuilding competitions. The usual diets of bodybuilders are composed of bland and plain foods that are often reduced to a handful of basic options.

- Turkey or chicken breast
- Grilled white fish
- Steamed veggies
- Rice cakes
- Brown rice
- Oatmeal
- Egg whites
- Protein shakes

These are usually referred to as "healthy" food, and there are many of them out there, all, dull and tasteless. By now you may see how eating these things every day, every week for months could end up really boring. This is one of the reasons why people quit their chosen diet or ditch away their fat loss goals totally. Surely, the conventional diets for body builders have been helping athletes to shred away fat for decades. But it is also true that these diets have also been making them miserable every time they take extreme diet.

The people who came up with the IIFYM dieting did so for the precise reason. They were weary of eating the same bland food when getting ready for a show. They were tired of avoiding the food they enjoy – the so called "unhealthy" food. Examples of unhealthy food are those that could satisfy our cravings but we are told to stay away from: fried chicken, French fries, ice cream, cookies, pop tarts, pizza, cheese cake, candy, Buffalo wings, and dough nuts.

The IIFYM Link

The first thing that people who want to start eating healthy is to think that they need to overhaul their diet. Usually, they think that they need to begin eating healthy food. Nevertheless, our society has cultured us about what is unhealthy and what is healthy.

This is not the case with IIFYM. Eating healthy food could specifically help you burn fat and lose weight, but there's no special link between weight loss and healthy food. The fat loss details are in the calorie count. Yes, calories. We are bombarded every day about watching your calories or counting your calories, but usually we ignore them. What you are about to read would shock most people. Consuming healthy foods haphazardly causes fat loss.

If you decide to clean up your diet and disregard calories, you instantly decrease your calorie intake. Removing sweets, sauces, and fried stuff will decrease your calories. There's no way around it. How much exactly? We can only guess. But certainly, less calories. The problem is that a significant drop could lead to metabolism restriction or at a minimum could decrease the metabolic capacity that makes stable and long-lasting weight loss much harder, and in some cases, could be impossible.

Because our everyday calorie intake affects how our bodies will look like, it is only reasonable that we go for healthy food to lose weight. However, eating healthy is not always the answer to fat loss. This is just a trick to help those who are not counting their calories and other macronutrients to lower them.

The main problem when we eat healthy food and we don't have any idea how much calories we are really taking, as well as how much our body needs, we end up becoming malnourished. We are basically starving ourselves, lining up our metabolism for a bounce back, which will certainly put you on extra pounds as soon as you return to your regular diet. In reality, eating normal often comes a lot sooner than we think when eating nothing but bland and mundane healthy foods.

For whatever reason, people think that they need to starve so they can lose weight. There are diet scams out there discrediting the importance of counting calories, and will sell you supplements or diet plans. Nonetheless, if they can convince you that counting calories instantly equates to starving yourself, then they can easily encourage you to buy the things they are selling.

Most people, regardless if they are couch potatoes or athletes know that they can get fat if they eat a lot. This is really a simple logic. Similarly, the more unhealthy food you eat, the faster you can get fat. The foundation of IIFYM diet lies in the middle of these two notions.

Based on the principles of IIFYM, it is fine to eat "unhealthy" food as long as you stay within your body's daily needed calorie intake. Remember, everyone is different. Our bodies are not the same, so we have different muscle mass, different metabolism, and many things that differentiate us from everyone else in this world. This is where IIFYM comes into the action. Instead of telling you how much calories you need according to your gender or according to your fitness goals, it examines every person individually and will recommend with high certainty how much calories to take.

There is no need to choose between that kale salad and that bacon pizza. You can even choose that ice cream instead of that oatmeal. You don't even need to count how much and how often you eat every day.

Devour the foods that you love, but keep within your body's macro nutrient need and shred off fat without the pain that most people link with dieting. A minimum of 15% decrease in calories is all you need in order to make your body a fat burning machine. This is the basic premise of IIFYM. Of course, there's more to it, but it is quite easy to understand:

- Determine the average amount that your calories burn every day
- Consume 10% to 20% less calories daily less than that number
- Divide the calories between protein, fat, and carbs, with enough water and fiber intake in a certain method, which preserves muscle and promotes weight loss without decreasing your daily energy

Finding the Balance

The main advantage of following the IIFYM diet is the flexibility and balance in your eating habit. A person who wants to add some foods that are more nutrient empty calorie could do that as long as he can still achieve the daily requirements and as long as they are still balancing their macronutrient percentage at every meal. Probably, this will take some time to absorb this concept, but it is really senseless to believe that a piece of muffin or enjoying a smoothie with your kids will sabotage all the work that you have been doing in the gym.

As a matter of fact, the humor is that most people who follow strictly to the idea of "healthy" eating will just give up after a short duration and will immerse on total binge eating, also known as "cheat" days. Truly, those binge eating will certainly wreak havoc on your body composition real fast.

Health and Body Composition are Not the Same Thing

Just because someone looks healthy, doesn't necessarily mean that he is healthy. Always remember that health is more than a slimmer waist or a six-pack. While the notion of IIFYM may appear as unhealthy, this is not actually the case. Once done appropriately,

IIFYM can fulfill all the requirements of a healthy and balanced diet.

It's not easy to change, especially eating habits. Most people feel safe in following what they know, but there are certain aspects in life that should be changed to reap the rewards. Experts recommend gradually easing your way into the nutritional change. The good thing about IIFYM is that it promotes flexible dieting, so there's definitely a learning curve, but once you become familiar, you can enjoy a diet that is just as effective as any popular diet regimen out there, if not more effective.

If you think about it, all the food that come naturally from nature are healthy, and all the food that are considered "unhealthy" are man-made such as sugar and processed food. All the food that are filled with minerals and nutrients can be harvested from nature. Even though IIFYM encourages diversity in the diet, you must make certain that your food options are coming from the proper sources. Choosing whole foods could easily enhance the health of a person. If you are eating the conventional highly-refined US diet, you are taking in 3000 calories without even knowing it. If you choose whole foods, you could get the same amount of nutrients and feel more satisfied with even half of the calories. It is food choices that are crucial in IIFYM.

Remember, IIFYM Is Not an Easy Way Out

At this point, you may feel that IIFYM is the easiest form of dieting regimen you can try. It really sounds good on paper, with the notion that you can have the ability to eat anything you like. Even though IIFYM allows dietary freedom, it still needs commitment. In reality, IIFYM dieting encourages you to be more precise. You don't just eat anything. You need to break down the calories into macros, which you will learn in the next Chapter.

Chapter 3 – Healthy Diet vs. IIFYM Diet Plan

Browse any typical bodybuilding website and you will stumble upon the same monotonous rubble, which now defines much of most people's diet.

Below is an example of a conventional "healthy" diet:

- Breakfast: 80 grams dry oats, six egg whites, 1 oz. almonds
- Pre-workout meal: 1 scoop of whey protein blended with 1 tbsp. of Flaxseed oil and 40 grams dry oats
- Post-workout meal: 2 scoops whey protein blended with 50 grams simple-carb solution such as pure dextrose or waxy maize
- Lunch: 1 cup steamed brown rice, 6 grams grilled chicken breast, and 2 cups sautéed broccoli
- Afternoon Snack: 1 scoop whey protein blended with 40 grams dry oats added with 1 tbsp. of Flaxseed oil
- Dinner: 1 scoop casein protein, 2 cups of sautéed asparagus plus 1 oz. mixed nuts

Overall Macronutrient Breakdown: 235 grams protein, 80 grams of fat, and 215 grams of carbohydrates.

Overall Calories: More or Less 2,520

Certainly, that's a healthy diet, but a diet composed of bland foods. This dieting approach usually leads to the loss of emotional pleasure, which must typically come from eating. It's unfortunate that most people would praise a person who is following this "healthy" diet, when in reality, it is too far from that.

Below is an example of an IIFYM diet plan, which also breaks down the same macronutrients as the diet above:

- Breakfast: 1 cup of cereal with milk, vegetable omelet, and 2 cups non-fat Greek yogurt mixed with ½ cup raspberries
- Lunch: 6 pieces chicken nuggets, 1 chicken sandwich, 1 small bowl of mixed fruits, 1 diet soda (medium)
- Post-workout Meal: 2 low-fat strawberry ice cream sandwiches, 1 cup low-fat cottage cheese blended with 1 oz. mixed nuts and a scoop of whey protein
- Dinner: 1 cup cooked spaghetti noodles relished with 12 oz. ground beef and marinara sauce

Overall Breakdown of Macronutrients: 215 grams carbohydrates, 235 grams protein, and 80 grams fat

Overall Calories: More or less 2520

Most people would love to follow the IIFYM diet plan. Take a look at the flexibility of this diet plan. It allows the person to eat what they want and take pleasure in small food cravings for the entire day.

Create Your Own IIFYM Meal Plan

A practical method of determining your macronutrient needs is to use a BMR calculator and the Harris-Benedict equation to figure out your everyday activity levels.

The link below will lead you to a comprehensive yet easy-to-use BMR calculator:

https://healthyeater.com/flexible-dieting-calculator/

For bodybuilders, it is ideal to consume around 1 gram of protein for every pound of lean body weight. When you have established your protein needs, you can move into your carb requirements, which should be based on the insulin sensitivity of your body.

Then after working on the carbohydrates and protein requirements, you can fill in the rest of your calorie requirements with fats.

For example, here's a meal work plan for an individual with 175 lbs of lean body mass and requires a 2750 calorie diet:

- Use the BMR Calorie Calculator to figure out the individual's calorie needs
- Establish your protein consumption at 1 gram per pound of lean body mass: 175 grams protein per day
- The person has high insulin sensitivity, so you can establish the carb consumption at 2 grams per pound lean body mass at 350 grams carbs per day (about 10% to 15% of this must be fiber).
- Because proteins and carbs contain 4 calories for every gram, than you can have (350+175) * 4: 2100 calories from carbs and proteins.
- Hence, the person's fat consumption will be sourced out from the remaining calories in order to achieve the target. So, 2750-2100 = 650 calories / 9 calories per gram of fat = more or less 72 grams of fat every day (and about 20% of these must be saturated fats)

If your goal is to lose fat, the general rule of thumb is to target an energy deficit of more or less 500 calories every day, most of which must come from decreased consumption of carbs. If you need to gain mass, target for an energy surplus of 300 to 500 calories daily.

Remember, these are only estimates, and you need to do some trial and error until you find what is suitable for your body.

Chapter 4 – Achieving Macronutrient Balance

An important principle that you must understand about IIFYM is that it doesn't deal with macronutrient balance across every meal. It is given that most fitness and health aficionados know that they must be taking a minimal amount of complete protein sources with every meal to provide enough increase in synthesizing muscle protein.

It is true that calories ultimately affects our whole system for gaining or losing weight, but certainly, there will be different effects on the body from a diet that significantly emphasizes consumption of macronutrient.

In order to demonstrate this example, take a closer look at two different caloric diet plans with similar macronutrient consumptions, which is more or less 2500 calories composed of 300 grams carbohydrates, 150 grams protein, and 75 to 80 grams of fat. However, they have different macronutrient balance for the entire day:

Meal Plan 1

(Balanced consumption with increased carbohydrates around the workout schedule)

Meal	Calories	Carbohydrates (g)	Protein (g)	Fat (g)
A	505	40	30	25
B (Pre-Workout)	575	80	30	15
C (Post-Workout)	390	80	25	10
D	450	50	30	15
E	600	50	40	15

Meal Plan 2

(Imbalanced consumption)

Meal	Calories	Carbohydrates (g)	Protein (g)	Fat (g)
A	480	5	110	5
B (Pre-Workout)	660	25	5	60
C (Post-Workout)	225	20	25	5
D	465	100	5	5
E	665	150	5	5

The caloric balances at every meal are really the same between these two meal plans. However, you can see the off-centered distribution of macros in Meal Plan 2. The second plan is loaded with carbohydrates while disregarding protein and fats. It is also nonsensical to consume a lot of carbohydrates on and then load up on fats during pre-training. In addition, the first meal of the day is basically excessive in protein. There are people who have even basic understanding of performance nutrition will never achieve balance their macronutrient consumption as described in Meal Plan 2.

This meal plan comparison is just to show the point that IIFY could be misinterpreted to mean that distributing macronutrients for the whole day is not important in trying to improve the body's nutritional composition. It may not play a primary role, but it still has a role to play nevertheless.

IIFYM Encourages People to Be Mindful yet Creative in Choosing Their Food

There are literally thousands of ways to eat a nutrient-rich and healthy diet that could improve both your physique and performance without compromising the quality and the flavor of your food. Never believe the nonsensical idea that you need to sacrifice the pleasure of eating so you can achieve your dream body.

IIFYM encourages people that they can still enjoy bacon, ice cream, cake, smoothies, pizza, cheese burger, and fries if they become creative and practice self-control into their everyday eating routine. If you really want to enjoy your favorite foods, all you need to do is to plan ahead and add those into your diet plan.

Conclusion

Thank you again for downloading this book!

I hope this book was able to help you get a better picture of what the IIFYM or flexible dieting system is.

The next step is to start taking action. Don't walk away from this book without starting to put these methods to use. Many people won't have even finished this book but you have, and now you have the power to start creating a clutter free lifestyle for now and forever.

I wish you the best of luck for your continued success!

Free Newsletter Signup

If you like my books and want to know when I launch a new one first, then please click the button below. It will take 2 seconds to fill out your email and I'll let you know when I launch a new book, often at a discount!

http://eepurl.com/bydh39

Did You Like *If It Fits Your Macros*?

Before you go, I'd like to say "thank you" for purchasing my book.

You could have picked from dozens of books about losing weight and building muscle but you took a chance to check out this one.

So a big thanks for downloading this book and reading all the way to the end.

Now I'd like ask for a *small* favor. Could you please take a minute or two and leave a review for this book on Amazon. This feedback will help me continue to write the kind of Kindle books that help you get results. And if you loved it, then please let me know :-)

Preview of 'The Gut Healing Protocol'

I've included the first section of my great guide to healing your gut. If this is something that might interest you then read on. Be sure to check out the other books I have on Kindle as well.

Chapter 1: Understanding Your Gut Flora

The human gut is home to approximately 100 trillion microorganisms with over 400 distinct bacterial species. But, despite the common conception of bacteria as causes of disease, the bacteria that make up your gut flora are beneficial and essential to your health. According to studies, your gut flora not only aids in digestion but also protects you from infections and disease by creating a barrier between your intestinal walls and bad bacteria, acting as your first line of defense. In fact, more than 75% of your immune system is made up of your gut flora.

A leaky gut, or gut dysbiosis, is a condition caused by worn out intestinal walls and weakened gut flora. This allows undigested food particles, chemicals and toxins to enter the bloodstream and trigger allergic reactions or other immune system problems. If left untreated, the immune system might become sensitive to certain foods and eventually result in food allergies. Leaky gut can also cause a variety of other problems such as diarrhea, constipation, rashes and bloating.

This book aims to help you remedy this situation and restore your gut health. However, before you can begin the process of healing your gut, it is important to clear some misconceptions first:

First of all, it is not only the food that you eat that affects your gut flora. Your good bacteria are heavily affected by your lifestyle. Factors such as sleep, exercise, stress levels and even your vitamin K status all have an effect on the health of your gut flora. So in the process of healing your gut, it is not enough to change only your eating habits, although it would play a large role in restoring the balance of your intestinal bacteria.

Second, healing your gut takes a lot of dedication. While the goal is to heal your gut in as little as a month, you will have to put in more effort to keep your gut healthy. Your intestinal bacteria can multiply and recover quickly, but it will take longer for them to adapt. It can also take a while before the effects of your new diet can be seen. But don't give up. One day isn't enough to heal your gut. Be patient and give it a few weeks. Your gut will be healthier and happier for it.

Third, elimination diets, or diets which only remove harmful food from your menu, such as wheat-free and gluten-free, aren't enough. Elimination diets are only one part of the process. It is important to avoid the foods which can cause inflammation and sensitivity of the gut to prevent further irritation. However, simply avoiding them does not heal the gut. The intestinal walls would still be exposed and food particles could still enter the bloodstream to cause allergic reactions. It is even more important to start eating healthy foods that will restore your gut flora to a working population, so it can resume its role in protecting you.

Fourth, don't worry about what you will be allowed to eat. Many people who set out to heal their gut give up out of the belief that it will limit their food options. But a healthy diet doesn't need to be bland. You will need to remove certain foods which can damage your gut from your diet. But that still leaves you with a variety of delicious and healthy foods to choose from. There are many great cookbooks out there which have menus that provide you with clean, nutritious and delicious meal options for a healthy gut.

Lastly, variety is good, but too much will not help. A lot of your gut bacteria are acquired from the foods which you regularly eat and this helps you digest these foods better. In a way, your gut flora learns from the good bacteria present in what you eat and this prevents you from developing allergic reactions to them. This means that the more familiar your body is to the food, the less likely it is to develop an allergic reaction. Give your gut time to learn by eating certain foods on a regular basis.

Click here to check out the rest of **The Gut Healing Protocol** on Amazon.

Or go to: **http://www.amazon.com/dp/B014X7CDXC**

Check Out My Other Books

Below you'll find some of my other popular books that are popular on Amazon and Kindle as well. Simply click on the links below to check them out. Alternatively, you can visit my author page on Amazon to see other work done by me.

Amazon Bestseller: Sugar Detox Diet: An Easy 10 Step Plan to Beat Sugar Cravings, Cure Carb Addiction, Lose Weight & Increase Your Energy

Amazon Bestseller: Low Carb, High Fat Diet: How to Lose Weight by Eating More

The Gut Healing Protocol: Reset Your Gut, Reduce Inflammation, Gain Energy and Feel Happier: 2nd Edition

The Ultimate Fat Burning Food Guide: Eat Foods That Boost Your Metabolism and Help Easily Burn Fat Away

The Truth About Cellulite: How to Get Rid of Cellulite Quickly, Naturally & Forever

How to Get Rid of Belly Fat: 7 Easy Ways to Lose Belly Fat Without Exercise!

How to Tone Your Body: 21 Days to a Total Body Transformation

How to Lose Weight Fast: 6 Essential Rules to Losing Weight Quickly and Easily

Fat Loss for Women: The Ultimate Fat Burning Bundle: Lose Weight Fast, Get Rid of Belly Fat and Tone Your Body

If the links do not work, for whatever reason, you can simply search for these titles on the Amazon website to find them.

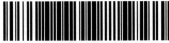

Made in the USA
Lexington, KY
13 April 2019